Leandro Lorenzi Rasia Dal Polo
Eduardo Galia Reston

Effect of Tooth Whitening and Two Adhesives

Leandro Lorenzi Rasia Dal Polo
Eduardo Galia Reston

Effect of Tooth Whitening and Two Adhesives

on the Shear Strength of Metal Brackets

ScienciaScripts

Imprint

Any brand names and product names mentioned in this book are subject to trademark, brand or patent protection and are trademarks or registered trademarks of their respective holders. The use of brand names, product names, common names, trade names, product descriptions etc. even without a particular marking in this work is in no way to be construed to mean that such names may be regarded as unrestricted in respect of trademark and brand protection legislation and could thus be used by anyone.

Cover image: www.ingimage.com

This book is a translation from the original published under ISBN 978-613-9-62418-8.

Publisher:
Sciencia Scripts
is a trademark of
Dodo Books Indian Ocean Ltd. and OmniScriptum S.R.L publishing group

120 High Road, East Finchley, London, N2 9ED, United Kingdom
Str. Armeneasca 28/1, office 1, Chisinau MD-2012, Republic of Moldova, Europe
Printed at: see last page
ISBN: 978-620-7-72645-5

SUMMARY

DEDICATORY

To Dona Lourdes, with nostalgia.

ACKNOWLEDGMENTS

To Prof. Dr. Eduardo Galia Reston for his safe, precise and objective guidance, without which this work would not have been possible.

To the mechanical testing laboratory at Ulbra/Canoas, in the person of technician Màrcio Moreira Allebrandt, who was always available and helpful.

To the statistician Prof. Dr. Màrio Wagner who made a lot of data and numbers inform something.

To the master's program in Dentistry at Ulbra/Canoas (management, professors and staff), which allowed a veteran student to venture back into the academic seas.

Knowledge makes the soul young and reduces the bitterness of old age.

Leonardo da Vinci

SUMMARY

The aim of this study was to compare the effects of two adhesives on the shear strength and adhesive remnant index (ARI) of orthodontic brackets bonded to bovine teeth bleached with 10% carbamide peroxide. The adhesives were Prime&Bond 2.1 (acetone-based) and Optibond S (ethanol-based). The brackets were bonded 24 hours after the end of bleaching. Eighty-two bovine incisors were used, divided into four groups: 1) non-bleached control group using Prime&Bond 2.1 adhesive; 2) non-bleached control group using Optibond S adhesive; 3) bleached experimental group using Prime&Bond 2.1 adhesive; and 4) bleached experimental group using Optibond S adhesive. ANOVA and Student-Newman-Keuls tests were applied to evaluate shear forces; and Kruskal-Wallis and Dunn's tests for ARI. The correlation between shear force and ARI was calculated using Spearman's correlation coefficient and its respective statistical significance using Student's t-test. The mean shear forces were 8.48 MPa ± 1.53 for the unbleached control group and Prime&Bond 2.1 adhesive; 12.21 MPa ± 2.37 for the unbleached control group and Optibond S adhesive; 8.89 MPa ± 2.16 for the bleached group and Prime&Bond 2.1 adhesive; and 10.41 MPa ± 2.73 for the bleached group and Optibond S adhesive. Statistically significant differences were found between all groups, except between the two groups that used Prime&Bond 2.1 adhesive. The ARI index showed a significant difference in the scores of the two bleached groups. All groups showed shear bond strength above the minimum acceptable clinical standard. The 24-hour interval between the end of home bleaching with 10% carbamide peroxide and the bonding of the brackets proved to be sufficient. The groups using Optibond S adhesive showed higher shear strength compared to the Prime&Bond 2.1 adhesive groups.

Keywords: Orthodontics. Whitening. Shear strength.

Tooth enamel.

1 - INTRODUCTION

Aesthetics are increasingly important in Western society. In this context, the smile is fundamental. Aligned, white teeth are the goal of many. Dentistry is faced with the challenge of solving an ever-increasing demand for orthodontic treatment and tooth whitening. Not infrequently, whitening and orthodontics are repeated throughout the patient's life. Often, the dental surgeon is faced with cases in which the logic of first orthodontic treatment and then whitening cannot be followed. Either because the patient comes to the orthodontist with the whitening done, or because they "demand" whitening beforehand, or because whitening becomes a tool for motivating and building patient loyalty in a competitive job market.

In the whitening of vital teeth, among the forms of whitening, either at home supervised by the dentist or in the office, two peroxides stand out: carbamide and hydrogen. The concentrations of these whitening gels and the time taken to apply them, in terms of number of sessions, length of sessions and days of application, differ greatly between authors.

Bonding the orthodontic appliance is a fundamental stage of treatment. The adhesion of the brackets must be high enough to resist spontaneous detachment, chewing forces and orthodontic mechanics (DELLA BONA, A.; GUIDA, L.A., 2014).

There is still controversy in the literature as to whether bleaching reduces the bond strength of the adhesives used to fix the brackets. Gungor et al. (2013), Nascimento et al. (2013), Scougall-Vilchis et al. (2011), Mullins et al. (2009), Patusco et al. (2009), Cacciafesta et al. (2006) and Prietsch et al. (2003) state that bleaching has a temporary effect on bond strength. Bishara et al. (2005) and Uysal et al. (2003) say that it does not. Kraether and Souza (2002) and Belo and Souza (2000) argue the opposite: bleaching increases adhesion.

Regarding the type of adhesive that should ideally be used after bleaching to bond the brackets, whether acetone-based or ethanol-based, there are differences of opinion. Authors such as Benni et al. (2004), Niat et al. (2012), Nour El-Din et al. (2006) and Swift et al. (1999) claim that acetone-based adhesives are superior, others such as Shinohara et al. (2004) and Sung et al. (1999) that ethanol-based adhesives are superior, and there are those who say that it doesn't matter (MONTALVAN, E. et al., 2006).

The methodology used in "in vitro" studies is totally different, making it difficult to compare results, despite the fact that there is an international technical standard guiding adhesion studies of dental materials. They differ from the type of tooth used, human or bovine, in the case of human, premolar and/or molar. In mechanical tests, the preparation of the specimens, the load used in the shear tests and the speed used in the machine differ profoundly from one work to another (FINNEMA, K.J. et al., 2010).

In this study, we followed the protocol recommended by the American Dental Association for supervised home whitening using 10% carbamide peroxide (ALQAHTANI, M. Q., 2014). The methodology used will be that of the international standard for testing adhesion to tooth structure (ISO/TS 11405, 2015), which accepts and encourages the use of bovine teeth, and establishes standards for preparing the specimens and carrying out the mechanical test.

The aim of this study was to establish the effect of bleaching and two adhesives, one ethanol-based and the other acetone-based, on the shear strength of metal orthodontic brackets. This was followed by an assessment of where adhesion failure occurred, using the Adhesive Remnant Index (ARI).

2 - LITERATURE REVIEW

Conservative aesthetic dentistry has grown dramatically. In the quest for beauty, orthodontics and whitening are in increasing demand. Whitening, among the options for improving dental appearance, is one of the most conservative and economical. We can classify whitening according to the vitality of darkened teeth into two broad classes: vital whitening and non-vital whitening (endodontically treated teeth). In vital whitening, we have in-office whitening, home whitening under the supervision of the dental surgeon and home whitening on free demand from the public. For home whitening of vital teeth, hydrogen peroxide (1.5% to 10%) and carbamide peroxide (5% to 30%) are used. For in-office whitening, 25% to 35% hydrogen peroxide is used, whether or not it is associated with the application of a light/heat source. It is controversial whether the application of a light/heat source speeds up the in-office whitening process (JOINER, A., 2006).

The whitening effect depends on the concentration of the whitening gel and the application time. It is an effective treatment, but not entirely predictable and responses are individual.

Vital whitening is recommended for cases of superficial pigmentation due to food and smoking and in mild cases of fluorosis and hypoplasia. In 2007, Knosel stated that whitening can be an effective solution for inactive white spots that occur after orthodontic treatment.

Among the adverse effects of whitening are gingival irritation, hypersensitivity, gastric irritation, nausea, loss of enamel structure, decreased adhesion of composites for restorations and bonding of brackets.

During whitening, pigmented foods and drinks, smoking, chlorhexidine mouthwashes and, if possible, medicines containing heavy metals should be avoided.

Carbamide peroxide at 10%, which is mainly used at home and was introduced by Haywood and Heymann in 1989, has been the whitening procedure that has grown in popularity due to its efficiency and simplicity.

According to Alqahtani, hydrogen peroxide, used in the dental office, has been associated with pre-neoplastic lesions, dental hypersensitivity, chronic inflammation, enamel demineralization and chemical irritation of the gums. Carbamide peroxide is more stable and the alkaline pH is safer for oral tissues. Carbamide peroxide breaks down intraorally into urea, ammonia, carbonic acid and hydrogen peroxide in low concentrations. This hydrogen peroxide is broken down into water and nascent oxygen, which quickly penetrate the porosity of the enamel, the organic matrix of this enamel and the dentin. The oxygen reacts quickly with the pigments, weakening the bonds between the chromogenic molecules and the organic matrix. These molecules are oxidized by the nascent oxygen and are broken down into smaller, less complex and lighter molecules. 10% carbamide peroxide has a concentration equivalent to 3-3.5% of hydrogen peroxide, and is therefore safer than the powerful 35% hydrogen peroxide of the more traditional concentrations used in dental practices. For this reason, carbamide peroxide is the safest alternative and is recommended by the American Dental Association ADA (ALQAHTANI, M. Q., 2014; MARTINS, M. M., 2008; HERINGER, T. P., 2007).

Various whitening systems have been used. Home-use carbamide peroxide, in the form of individual trays, has been used in the most varied concentrations (10 to 45%), lasting 4 to 8 hours for 5 to 14 consecutive days (BENNI, D. et al., 2014; GUNGOR, A.Y. et al., 2013; NIAT, A. B. et al., 2012; PHAN, X. et al., 2012; SCOUGALL-VILCHIS, A. B. et al., 2012), 2013; NIAT, A. B. et al., 2012; PHAN, X. et al., 2012; SCOUGALL-VILCHIS, R. J. et al., 2011; PATUSCO, V.C. et al., 2009; UYSAL, T. & SISMAN, A., 2008; BULUT, H. et al., 2006; NOUR EL-DIN, et al., 2006; BISHARA, S. E. et al., 2005; SUNG, E. C. et al., 1999). Hydrogen peroxide is generally the choice for in-office whitening, with concentrations ranging from 15-45%, which may or may not be activated by a heat and/or light source, the number of sessions varying from 1 to 3 and the application time from 15 minutes to 1 hour per appointment (YADAV, D. et al., 2015; GUNGOR, A.Y. et al., 2013; NASCIMENTO, G.C.R. et al., 2013; SCOUGALL- VILCHIS, R. J. et al., 2011; MULLINS, A. et al., 2009; PATUSCO, V.C. et al., 2009; TUKKAHRAMAN, H. et al.., 2007; MONTALVAN, E. et al., 2006; NOUR EL-DIN, et al., 2006; CACCIAFESTA, V. et al., 2006; BISHARA, S. E. et al., 2005; UYSAL, T. et al., 2003). Studies shown in tables 1, 2 and 3, respectively on pages 24, 25 and 26.

Efficient orthodontic treatment requires proper bonding of the brackets to the tooth enamel. Bleaching alters the roughness of the enamel surface and increases its porosity due to mineral loss. This surface alteration can affect the quality of bonding by reducing the number and length of resin tags. Oxygen plays an antagonistic role: on the one hand it is the active ingredient in whitening, on the other it is an inhibitor of polymerization. The effect of carbamide peroxide on the bonding strength of brackets to enamel is controversial. One of the hypotheses to explain a possible reduction in post-bleaching bond strengths is the presence of residual oxygen which inhibits polymerization. There is obviously interest in determining whether changes in the enamel surface can result in changes in the adhesive characteristics of bonding materials. Gungor et al. (2013), Nascimento et al. (2013), Scougall-Vilchis et al. (2011), Mullins et al. (2009), Patusco et al. (2009), Cacciafesta et al. (2006) and Prietsch et al. (2003) have reported a severe decrease in the bond strengths of composites to bleached enamel when compared to unbleached enamel. Authors such as Bishara et al. (2005) and Uysal et al. (2003) found no effect on the bond strengths of orthodontic brackets to bleached enamel when compared to unbleached enamel. While Belo and Souza (2000) observed a significant increase in the bond strengths of brackets bonded with modified glass ionomer after bleaching with 10% carbamide peroxide due to surface erosion of the enamel caused by the bleaching gel. Kraether and Souza (2002) also demonstrated that the action of 10% carbamide peroxide, in vitro, promoted a significant increase in the bond strength of the resin to the enamel when bonding brackets.

The waiting time, and even the need to wait, between the end of bleaching and the bonding of the brackets is also controversial. The following studies ranged from 30 minutes (NASCIMENTO, G.C.R. et al., 2013) to 30 days (UYSAL, T. & SISMAN, A., 2008), and could be 24 hours, two days, one, two, three or four weeks (GUNGOR, A.Y. et al., 2013; PHAN, X. et al., 2012; SCOUGALL-VILCHIS, R. J. et al., 2011; MULLINS, A. et al., 2009; PATUSCO, V.C. et al., 2009; TUKKAHRAMAN, H. et al., 2007; BISHARA, S. E. et al., 2005). The articles by Yadav et al. (2015), Bulut et al. (2006), Cacciafesta et al. (2006) state that bonding took place immediately after bleaching, but did not specify this time (tables 1 and 2, pages 24 and 25). Mullins et al. (2009) therefore recommend waiting 2 to 3 weeks between bleaching and bonding. Gungor et al. (2013) recommend waiting until orthodontic treatment is complete before carrying out whitening. Nascimento et al. (2013) recommend waiting three weeks before bonding brackets in the case of in-office whitening.

Some experiments such as those by Benni et al. (2014), Niat et al. (2012), Nour El-Din et al. (2006) and Swift et al. (1999) have shown that the use of an acetone-based adhesive can eliminate the need to wait some time before working on bleached enamel. This is because acetone acts as a "moisture sequestrator", known as the "water chaser" effect, which displaces water from the tooth surface. Acetone is also the best solvent for "loading" the resin into the etched tooth surface, forming longer, more structured "tags". But there is controversy about this.

Sung et al. (1999) evaluated "in vitro" the effect of three adhesive agents: All Bond 2 (acetone-based adhesive), Optibond (ethanol-based) and One Step (acetone-based). The composite resin used for the 3 groups was Herculite in the form of "stubs" bonded to the enamel. For Optibond (ethanol-based), there was no statistically significant difference between the control and bleached groups in terms of shear forces. However, in bleached enamel bonded with All Bond 2 or One Step (acetone-based adhesives), the shear forces were significantly lower than in the control group. Ethanol would interact with residual oxygen and minimize the inhibitory effect of the bleaching process on the formation of resin tags. They concluded that ethanol-based adhesives can be used immediately after bleaching. However, these authors waited 5 days after bleaching before carrying out the restorative procedure. Shinohara et al. (2004) also observed that ethanol-based adhesives and water-based adhesives showed significantly higher shear forces than acetone-based adhesives, table 4 on page 27.

Montalvan et al. (2006) concluded that shear forces did not differ between acetone-based and ethanol-based adhesives 24 hours after bleaching with 35% hydrogen peroxide on human molars and premolars, table 3 on page 26.

The methodology used in mechanical tests differs widely, making it difficult to compare the results obtained (FINNEMA, K.J. et al., 2010; FARRET, M.M. et al., 2010). There is no standardization, although there is an international technical standard ISO/TS 11405 (2015) for testing adhesion to tooth structure. The choice of mechanical shear tests is justified by the fact that they best simulate chewing forces (YADALA, C. et al., 2015; YADAV, D. et al., 2015; BENNI, D. et al., 2014; GUNGOR, A.Y. et al.,2013; NASCIMENTO, G.C.R. et al., 2013; PHAN, X. et al., 2012; NIAT, A. B. et al., 2012; SCOUGALL-VILCHIS, R. J. et al., 2011; PATUSCO, V.C. et al., 2009; UYSAL, T. & SISMAN, A., 2008; TUKKAHRAMAN, H. et al., 2007; BULUT, H. et al., 2006; CACCIAFESTA, V. et al., 2006; MONTALVAN, E. et al., 2006; NOUR EL-DIN, et al., 2006; BISHARA, S. E. el al., 2005; SHINOHARA, M. S. et al., 2004; SWIFT, E. J. et al., 1999). The chisel application speed in the test varied from 0.5 mm per minute (BENNI, D. et al., 2014; GUNGOR, A.Y. et al.,2013; NASCIMENTO, G.C.R. et al., 2013; PHAN, X. et al.,2012; SCOUGALL-VILCHIS, R. J. et al., 2011; PATUSCO, V.C. et al., 2009; UYSAL, T. & SISMAN, A., 2008; TUKKAHRAMAN, H. et al., 2007; NOUR EL-DIN, et al., 2006; SHINOHARA, M. S. et al., 2004); 1mm per minute (YADALA, C. et al., 2015; YADAV, D. et al., 2015; NIAT, A. B. et al., 2012; BULUT, H. et al., 2006; CACCIAFESTA, V. et al., 2006); 5 mm per minute (BISHARA, S. E. et al., 2005; SWIFT, E. J. et al., 1999); 0.05 inches per minute (SUNG, E. C. et al., 1999). The load cell was 50Kg (PATUSCO, V.C. et al., 2009); 1000 Newtons (YADAV, D. et al.,2015; PHAN, X. et al., 2012) and they did not report it (YADALA, C. et al., 2015; GUNGOR, BENNI, D. et al., 2014; A.Y. et al.,2013; NASCIMENTO, G.C.R. et al., 2013; NIAT, A. B. et al., 2012; SCOUGALL-VILCHIS, R. J. et al., 2011; UYSAL, T. & SISMAN, A., 2008; TUKKAHRAMAN, H. et al., 2007; BULUT, H. et al., 2006; CACCIAFESTA, V. et al., 2006; MONTALVAN, E. et al., 2006; NOUR EL-DIN, et al., 2006; BISHARA, S. E. el al., 2005; SHINOHARA, M. S. et al., 2004; SWIFT, E. J. et al., 2009), as seen in tables 1,2, 3 and 4 on pages 24, 25, 26 and 27.

In order to evaluate where the adhesion failure occurred, whether on the enamel surface, inherent to the resin itself or in the retentive area of the bracket, Yadala et al. (2015), Gungor et al. (2013), Nascimento et al. (2013), Phan et al. (2012), Scougall-Vilchis et al. (2011), Mullins et al. (2009), Patusco et al. (2009), Uysal and Sisman (2008), Tukkahraman et al. (2007), Bulut et al. (2006), Cacciafesta et al. (2006) and Uysal et al. (2003) used the Adhesive Remnant Index (ARI) recommended by Artun and Bergland in 1984, tables 1 and 2, pages 24 and 25. This index establishes scores from 0 to 3 according to the amount of resin remaining on the enamel surface after removing the brackets. Where: 0 - no resin on the enamel;

1   - less than 50% of the resin remaining in the enamel;

2   - more than 50% of the resin remaining in the enamel;

3   - 100% resin remaining on the enamel after peeling.

Nakamichi et al. (1983) evaluated a substitute for human teeth in adhesion tests. The adhesion of glass ionomer cement, zinc phosphate, polycarboxylate and two composite resins (Adaptic and Clearfil) to bovine enamel and dentin was compared to human teeth. They observed that the strength of adhesion to enamel showed no statistically significant difference between bovine and human teeth, although the average values were lower in the former.

Tables 1, 2, 3 and 4 (pages 24, 25, 26 and 27) show that Scougall-Vilchis et al. (2011), Nour El-Din et al. (2006), Cacciafesta et al. (2006), Shinohara et al. (2004) and Swift et al. (1999) opted to use bovine teeth in their studies. Other authors used human teeth, ranging from molars (PHAN et al., 2012; BISHARA et al., 2005; SUNG et al., 1999) to premolars (YADALA et al., 2015; YADAV et al., 2015; GUNGOR et al., 2013; NASCIMENTO et al., 2013; NIAT et al., 2012; PATUSCO et al., 2009; UYSAL et al., 2008; TUKKAHRAMAN et al. 2007; BULUT et al., 2006; UYSAL et al.,2003). Montalvan et al. (2006) used a sample of molars and premolars indistinctly. Benni et al. (2014) used a sample of 120 human incisors.

The ideal tooth for adhesion testing is the human incisor, which allows the base of the bracket to be adapted to the flat enamel surface with the minimum amount of bonding material. The difficulty of obtaining these teeth in our country makes it impossible to use them. In our literature review, only the Indian study by Benni et al. (2014) used them. The most easily obtained human teeth, premolars and especially third molars, show great anatomical variability. This results in a greater thickness of bonding resin between the enamel and the base of the bracket, which can lead to bonding bias. The ISO/TS 11405 (2015) technical standard for testing adhesion to tooth structure recommends the use of bovine incisors and establishes standards for their preparation.

Table 1 - Data on the review articles and their results

Author	Objective	Sample	Whitening	Interval whitening gluing	Essay Mechanic	Speed	Cell Load	ARI	Results
Yadav 2015 J. Orthod. Science	To evaluate the effects of antioxidant agents (sodium ascorbate, tocopherol acetate and retinol acetate) on shear forces in brackets bonded to bleached teeth.	100 human MPs divided into 5 groups	PH at 35% for 16 min, activated by light	Immediately	Shearing	1 mm/min	1000N	N	Bleaching alone reduces shear forces. Antioxidants reverse this reduction.
Yadala 2015 J. Internat. Oral Health	Comparing shear forces and ARI of 3 self-conditioning adhesives **Adper PromtXeno III Transbond Plus**	60 human MPs divided into 4 groups	Not realized	Not applicable	Mento shears	1 mm/min	No information	S	There was no significant difference between the groups
Gungor 2013 AngleOrth	To evaluate the effects of whitening (home and office) on the bonding of brackets	45 MPs divided into 3 groups	Consult: PH 15% - 1 hour on 3 consecutive days. Homemade: PC 10% - 8h/day for 3 weeks	4 weeks	Shearing	0.5 mm/min	No information.	S	Both types of bleaching affected the shear forces, but the in-office bleaching was more adverse.
Birth 2013 Korean J Orthod	Evaluate the shear forces in post-bleaching bonded brackets at 4 intervals.	90 human MPs divided into 9 groups	Homemade: PH at 7.5% - 1h/day for 3 weeks. Consult: PH at 35% - 15 min X 3	30 minutes 1 day 2 weeks 3 weeks	Shearing	0.5 mm/min	No Inform.	S	All the bleached groups had reduced shear forces. The values returned to normal after 3 weeks.
Phan 2012 AngleOrth.	Evaluate the effects of home whitening + consultation on bonding with **ProSeal** fluoride-releasing sealant compared to TransBond	160 molars divided into 4 groups	One session in consultation. With PC at 45% for 30 minutes + 5 home applications of PC at 20% for 6 hours	2 weeks	Shearing	0.5 mm/min	1000N	S	Both sealants are good bonding options, although **ProSeal** has demonstrated lower shear forces.
Scougall-Vilchis 2011 AngleOrth.	Comparing 4 whitening systems on shear forces in brackets	150 bovine teeth divided into 5 groups	1.PH 38% for 15 min 2.PC 10% - 8 hrs/day for 7 days 3. RBCH - **Beauty coat** 4. RBCH - **White coat**	24 hours	Shearing	0.5 mm/min	No information	S	Home and office bleaching significantly reduced shear forces. RBCH did not affect these forces.
Mullins 2009	Evaluate the survival rate of "in vivo" brachytes	38 patients	Consult: PH 38% - 2 cycles of 15 min.	24 hours 3 weeks	Not applicable	Not applicable	Not applicable	S	The survival rate was higher for unbleached teeth. Among the bleached teeth, it was higher when

Author	Objective	Sample	Whitening	Interval whitening gluing	Essay Mechanic	Speed	Cell Load	ARI	Results
AngleOrth.									waiting 3 weeks.
Patusco 2009 AngleOrth.	To evaluate the effects of whitening (home and office) on the bonding of brackets	45 MPs divided into 3 groups	Homemade: PC 10% - 4h/day for 14 days Consult: PH 35% - 6 minutes X 4	24 hours	Shearing	0.5 mm/min	50 Kg	S	There was no difference between the control group and home whitening. However, in-office whitening showed lower values.

Caption - PM: premolars; PH: hydrogen peroxide; PC: carbamide peroxide; ARI: adhesive remnant index; Y: yes; N: no.

Table 2 - Data on the review articles and their results

Author	Objective	Sample	Whitening	Interval whitening gluing	Essay Mechanic	Speed	Cell Load	ARI	Results
Uysal 2008 Angle orth.	Evaluate the effects of bleaching on shear forces and ARI in brackets bonded with Transbond self-conditioning	60 human MPs divided into 3 groups	Perox. carbamide 16% for 4 hours on 10 consecutive days	In two stages: immediately and after 30 days	Shearing	0.5 mm/min	No information	S	Whitening immediately before bonding significantly reduces shear forces.
Turkkahram 2007 Angle Orth.	Evaluate the effects of bleaching and Ultraez desensitizer on the shear forces of brackets	48 human MPs divided into 4 groups	Perox. hydrog. 35% applied for 15 min X 2 at the same appointment	2 days	Shearing	0.5 mm/min	No information	S	Whitening and Ultraez (desensitizer based on Nitrate) reduced the shear forces significance
Bulut 2006 HELP	Effect of 10% sodium ascorbate antioxidant on bonding	80 human MPs	Homemade: PC 10% - 8 hours a day for 7 days	Immediately and one week	Shearing	1 mm/min	No Inform	S	Sodium ascorbate is an alternative to waiting between bleaching and bonding
Bishara 2005 AJODO	To evaluate the effects of whitening (home and office) on the bonding of brackets	75 human molars	Homemade: PC 10% - 6 h/day for 14 days. Office: PH. 25% - 20 min X 2	7 and 14 days	Shearing	5 mm/min	I don't know.	N	No difference between groups
Cacciafesta 2005 AJODO	Effect of bleaching on bonding of **Fuji Ortho** brackets	45 bovine incisors divided into 3 groups	Consult:PH 35% - 20 min X 2	Immediately and one week	Shearing	1 mm/min	No Inform.	S	Bleaching decreased the bond strengths of the **Fuji Ortho** Cement
Uysal 2003 AJO-DO	Evaluate the effects of bleaching on shear forces and ARI at two time points	60 human MPs divided into 3 groups	Peroxide hydrogen 35% activated by light	In two stages: immediately and after 30 days	Shearing	0.5 mm/min	No information	S	There was no significant difference between the groups.

Caption - PM: premolars; PH: hydrogen peroxide; PC: carbamide peroxide; ARI: adhesive remnant index; Y: yes; N: no.

Table 3 - Data on the review articles and their results

Author	Objective	Sample	Whitening	Interval whitening gluing	Essay Mechanic	Speed	Cell Load	Results
Benni 2014	To evaluate the effects of	120 human incisors	Homemade:	Immediately	Shearing	0,5 mm/min	Not informed	Acetone-based adhesives

Author	Objective	Sample	Whitening	Interval whitening gluing	Essay Mechanic	Speed	Cell Load	Results
Indian Society Pedodontics Preventive Dentistry	ethanol-based adhesives **Clearfill and Adpter** and acetone-based adhesives **Prime and Bond and One Step** on shear forces in composites applied to bleached enamel.	divided into 8 groups of 15	10% PC for 6 h/day for 5 days					showed higher shear forces, but this difference was not statistically significant
Niat 2012 J Adhes. Dent	To evaluate the effect of drying agents (70% alcohol and acetone) and different adhesives (acetone and ethanol-based) on the bond strengths of composite resins immediately after bleaching.	60 human premolars divided into three groups according to the "drying" agent used: alcohol 70, acetone and distilled water. Each group was subdivided into two according to the adhesive used: ethanol-based **Single Bond** and acetone-based **One Step**	Homemade: PC at 15% for 6 hours for five consecutive days	24 hours	Shearing	1 mm/min	Not informed	The acetone-based adhesive (**One Step**) provided higher bond strengths than the ethanol-based adhesive (**Single Bond**)
Montalvan 2006 Pediatric Dentistry.	Evaluate the effects of ethanol-based **Bond 1 C&P** and acetone-based **Bond 1** adhesives on shear forces in composites applied to bleached enamel	40 human molars and PMs divided into 4 groups	Consulting room: PH at 35% for 15 minutes activated by light. Repeated a second time	24 hours	Shearing	Not informed	No Inform	Shear forces were significantly lower in bleached teeth compared to unbleached teeth. However, these forces did not differ between the acetone- and ethanol-based adhesives.
Nour El-Din 2006 Operative Dentistry	To evaluate the shear forces when **Single Bond** ethanol-based and **One Step** acetone-based adhesives were used immediately after bleaching.	72 bovine incisors divided into 3 groups according to the bleaching used	Clinic: PH at 38% for 30 mins Homemade: PC at 10% for 6h/day for 5 days	24 hours	Shearing	0,5 mm/min	I don't know.	**One Step** (acetone) showed higher shear strengths than **Single Bond** (ethanol), but the difference was not statistically significant.

Caption - PM: premolars; PH: hydrogen peroxide; PC: carbamide peroxide; ARI: adhesive remnant index.

Table 4 - Data on the review articles and their results

Author	Objective	Sample	Whitening	Interval whitening gluing	Essay Mechanic	Speed	Cell Load	Results
Shinohara 2004 J Adhes Dent	To evaluate the effect of three different adhesives: **Single Bond** (ethanol/water solvent), **Prime & Bond NT**	270 bovine teeth were divided into three groups according to the bleaching agent used (sodium	Non-vital whitening in two forms: **sodium perborate**	7 days	Shearing	0.5 mm/min	No inform	Bleaching treatment on enamel and dentin reduced bond strengths, regardless of the type of adhesive used. However, **Single Bond**

	(acetone solvent) and **Clearfil** (water solvent) on the shear strength of composite resin after bleaching.	perborate, PC and control). Each group was divided into six subgroups of 15 each, according to the bonding substrate (enamel or dentin) and the adhesive used	paste + water and 37% **PC.** Renewed weekly for 3 weeks.					(ethanol/water) and **Clearfil** (water) showed significantly higher shear forces than **Prime & Bond NT** (acetone) for both bleached and unbleached dental tissues.
Sung 1999 J. Prosthetic dentistry	To evaluate the effect of three adhesive agents: **All Bond 2** (based on acetone), **Optibond** (ethanol) and **One Step** (acetone) on the shear forces in bleached enamel	24 human molars	10% PC was applied once a day for six hours for five consecutive days	5 days	Shearing	0,05 inches/min	No inform	For **Optibond** (ethanol-based), there was no statistically significant difference between the bleached and control groups in terms of shear forces. However, in bleached enamel bonded with **All Bond 2** or **One Step** (acetone base), the shear forces were significantly lower than in the control group.
Swift 1999 J Esthetic Dentistry	To evaluate the shear forces of six single-bottle adhesives applied to wet enamel.	105 bovine incisors divided into 7 groups (**OneStep** acetone, **OptiBond Solo** ethanol, **Prime & Bond 2.1** acetone, **Syntac SingleComponent** water, **Single Bond** ethanol/water, **Tenure Quik** acetone) and the control **Scotchbond** water	Not realized	Not applicable	Shearing	5 mm/min	No Inform	All the single-bottle adhesives achieved a shear force of over 21 MPa. **Prime&Bond 2.1** (acetone-based) had a much higher average shear force than the others (29.6 MPa).

Caption - PM: premolars; PH: hydrogen peroxide; PC: carbamide peroxide; ARI: adhesive remnant index.

3 - PROPOSAL

To evaluate the influence of 10% carbamide peroxide bleaching and two adhesives, one acetone-based and the other ethanol-based, on the adhesion of metal orthodontic brackets:

1.   shear strength on a universal testing machine

2.   the areas of adhesive failure using the Adhesive Remnant Index (ARI).

4 - MATERIAL AND METHODS

4.1   - Sample: 90 bovine incisors were obtained from Frigorifico Bravo Ltda, Ana Rech, Caxias do Sul-RS. Eight were discarded because of enamel defects on the buccal side of the crown, fractures or abrasions, leaving 82.

The teeth were randomly divided into the following groups:

Group 1. Control group in which no bleaching was carried out. Stored in artificial saliva for 15 days. After this period, the bracket was bonded with acetone-based adhesive (Prime & Bond 2.1) and Transbond XT resin. Again stored in artificial saliva until the shear test was carried out.

Group 2. Control group in which no bleaching was carried out. Stored in artificial saliva for 15 days. After this period, the bracket was bonded with ethanol-based adhesive (Optibond S) and Transbond XT resin. Again stored in artificial saliva until the shear test was carried out.

Group 3. Experimental group in which bleaching was carried out with 10% carbamide peroxide (Opalescence) in daily cycles of 8 hours for 14 consecutive days. Twenty-four hours after the last bleaching session, the bracket was bonded with acetone-based adhesive (Prime & Bond 2.1) and Transbond XT resin. This 24-hour period is in line with studies by Martins (2008), Dishmann et al. (1994) and Titley et al. (1992). These authors state that this is enough time for the residual oxygen present in the enamel to be released after bleaching. Again stored in artificial saliva until the shear test.

Group 4. Experimental group in which bleaching was carried out with 10% carbamide peroxide (Opalescence) in daily cycles of 8 hours for 14 consecutive days. Twenty-four hours after the last bleaching session, the bracket was bonded with ethanol-based adhesive (Optibond S) and Transbond XT resin. Again stored in artificial saliva until the shear test was carried out (table 5, page 32).

Table 5 - Sample groups

Group	Whitening	Sticker	Sample number
1	No	Prime & Bond 2.1	20

2	No	Optibond S	21
3	Yes	Prime & Bond 2.1	20
4	Yes	Optibond S	21

4.2 - Preparation of the specimens - In all the steps involved in preparing and handling the specimens, the operator wore PPE (personal protective equipment - apron, mask, goggles and gloves). After extraction and evaluation, the remaining 82 teeth were brushed under running water and stored in 0.1% thymol for a week, for antiseptic purposes. They were then stored in distilled water until the specimens were prepared.

The teeth had their crowns separated from the roots using a carborundum disk (KG Sorensen, Cotia, SP, Brazil) at the cervical level (figure 1, page 32).

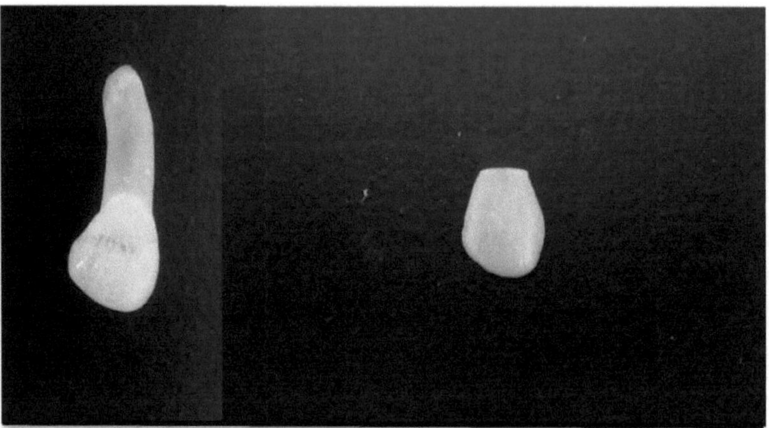

Figure 1 - Whole bovine incisor on the left and cut at the cervical level on the right.

Each crown was then placed in a PVC (polyvinyl chloride) ring 25 mm in diameter and 15 mm high (Tigre, Joinville, SC, Brazil) (figure 2, page 33).

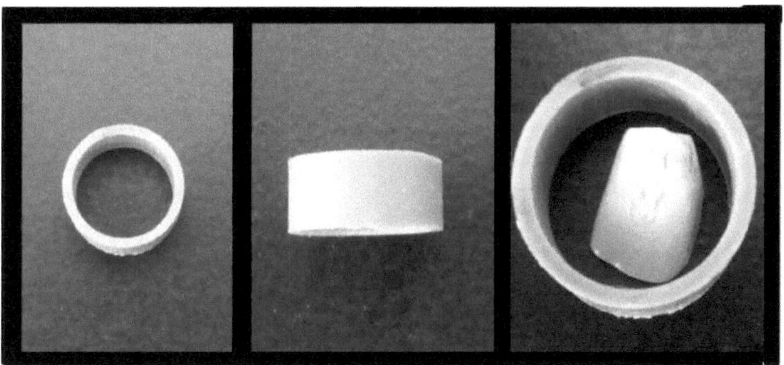

Figure 2 - PVC ring on the left and center, crown included on the right.

This ring was supported on a glass plate and the buccal side of the tooth crown was facing this plate. Self-curing acrylic resin (Jet Clàssico, Sao Paulo, SP, Brazil) was then poured in, completely filling the ring. A second plate was placed on top of the ring to create a flat, smooth surface (figure 3, page 33). It was left to polymerize for 24 hours.

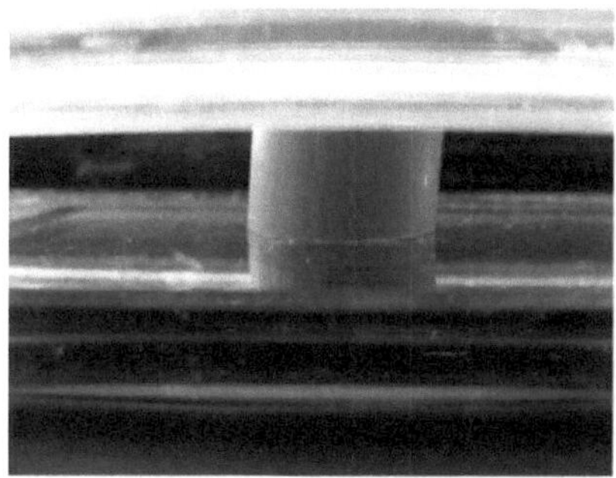

Figure 3 - PVC ring between two glass plates.

The side of the ring with the vestibular face of the crown was exposed by the action of an orbital sander (DeWalt, Uberaba, MG, Brazil), using the 120, 400 and 600 water sandpaper sequence (Norton, Guarulhos, SP, Brazil) for 15 seconds each, according to ISO/TS 11405:2015. Once sanding was complete, the surface of the exposed crown was evaluated under a 10X magnifying glass. There should be a flat area of enamel exposed, compatible with the base of the bracket that would be bonded (figure 4, page 34). If dentin was exposed, the specimen was discarded.

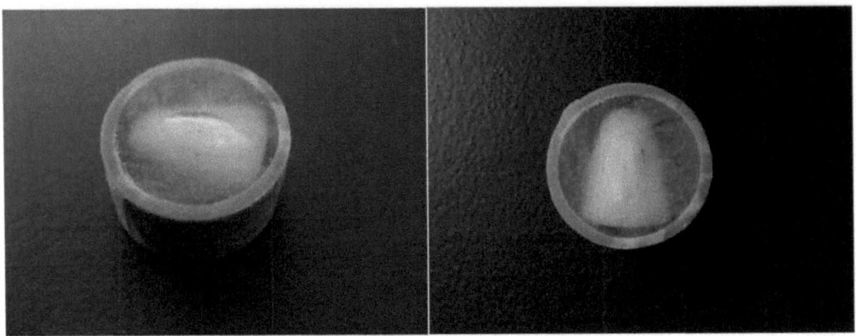

Figure 4 - Exposed, flat area of enamel compatible with the base of the bracket.

4.3   - Whitening - Whitening was carried out on 41 specimens, groups 3 and 4, with 10% carbamide peroxide for home use Opalescence PF Regular (Ultradent, South Jordan, UT, USA), the only one recommended by the American Dental Association (OPALESCENCE, 2016) (figure 5, page 34) and (table 6, page 37). The whitening gel was applied to the polished and flattened buccal surface in daily 8-hour cycles over 14 consecutive days. At the end of each cycle, the specimens were rinsed thoroughly and stored in artificial saliva. Once bleaching was complete, a 24-hour wait was made and the brackets were bonded.

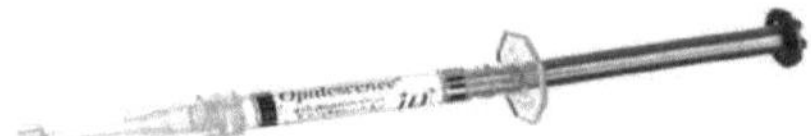

Figure 5 - Opalescence syringe

4.4   - Bracket bonding - The buccal surface was prophylaxed with pumice stone (SS White, Rio de Janeiro, RJ, Brazil) using a Robison brush (Microdont, Sao Paulo, SP, Brazil) at low speed for 15 seconds, then washed with a jet of water and dried with an air jet, free from oil and moisture.

The 37% phosphoric acid etchant (Dentisply Caulk, Milford, DE, USA) commonly used in all groups was applied for 15 seconds with immediate washing and drying with moisture- and oil-free water and air jets for 15 seconds. The adhesive was applied to the conditioned surface using a microbrush applicator (KG Sorensen, Cotia, SP, Brazil) with a light brushing movement for 15 seconds. Air jet applied for 3 seconds to reduce thickness. Light-cured for 20 seconds. The acetone-based adhesive for groups 1 and 3 was Prime & Bond 2.1 (Dentisply Caulk, Milford, DE, USA) and the ethanol-based adhesive for groups 2 and 4 was Optibond S (Kerr, Orange, CA, USA) (figure 6, page 35).

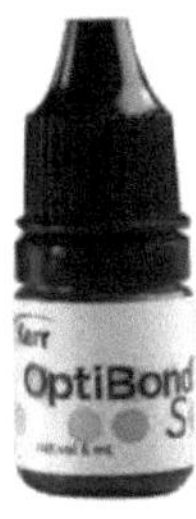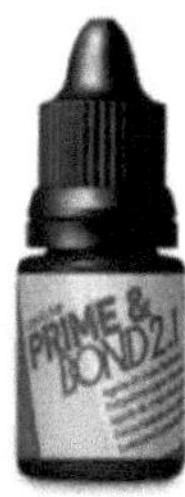

Figure 6 - Optibond S adhesive and Prime & Bond 2.1.

The resin was positioned at the base of the bracket with a 3S sculptor (Duflex, Juiz de Fora, MG, Brazil) and this was brought to the tooth with orthodontic tweezers (Morelli, Sorocaba, SP, Brazil). The resin used in all groups was Transbond XT (3M Unitek, Monrovia, CA, USA) (figure 7, page 35).

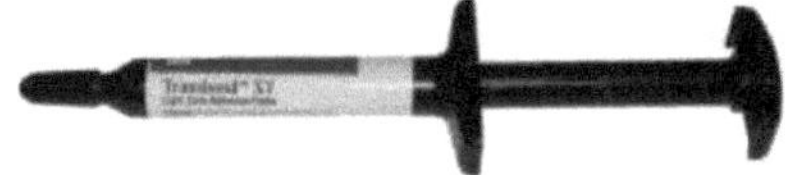

Figure 7 - Transbond XT

Edgewise 022X.028 upper central incisor metal brackets were used, reference 204-101 (3M Abzil, Sâo José do Rio Preto, SP, Brazil). Made from 17/4 steel, with 80 micron mesh spacing and a base area of 15.13 mm^2 . The bracket was positioned in the center of the tooth crown (figure 8, page 36). Light pressure was applied to the bracket. Excess resin was removed with an exploratory probe (Duflex, Juiz de Fora, MG, Brazil). The resin was polymerized for a total of 40 seconds, 20 per mesial and 20 per distal, using a 500 nm, 75 W light-curing device, model Optilight Plus (Gnatus, Ribeirâo Preto, SP, Brazil). The teeth were then stored in artificial saliva until the shear test.

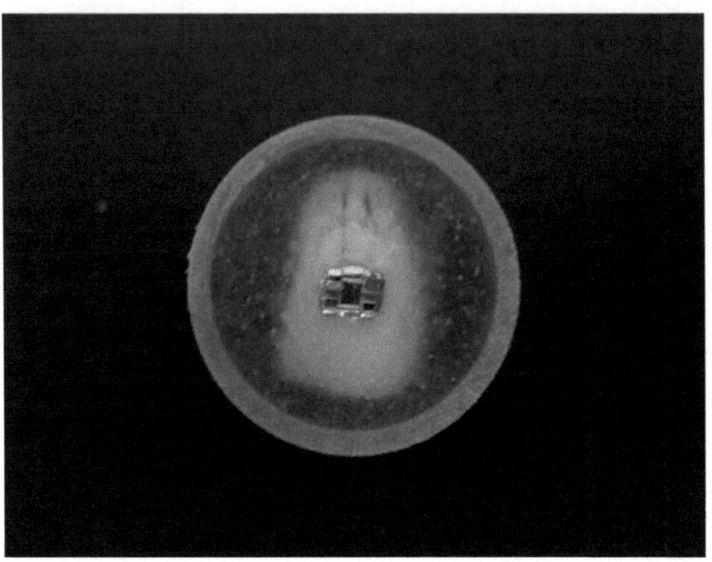

Figure 8 - Bracket glued to the center of the crown

Table 6 - Presentation of materials.

Material	Manufacturer	Composition	Lot
Opalescence PF Regular	Ultradent	10% carbamide peroxide, fluorine, potassium nitrate	D00Y1
37% phosphoric acid	Dentisply	Phosphoric acid; Surfactant; Aerosil 200; Deionized water and Pigment.	525532D
Optibond S	Kerr	BIS-GMA, HEMA, GDM, GPDM, ethanol, silica, barium glass, camphorquinone.	5819163
Prime&Bond 2.1	Dentisply	UDMA Resin; Penta; R5-62-1 Resin; Camphorquinone; EDAB (Ethyl Dimethyl Aminobenzoate); BHT (Butyl Hydroxytoluene); Bisphenol A dimethacrylate Pò; Cetylamine Fluoride and Acetone PA.	179474I
Transbond XT	3M Unitek	Silica, Bis- GMA, silane, n-dimethylbenzocaine, hexa-fluoro-phosphate	N740303
Edgewise brackets Central Incisor	3M Abzil	steel 17/4	1618700175

Upper .022X.028			

4.5 - Strength tests - were carried out at the Mechanical Testing Laboratory of the Lutheran University of Brazil (Ulbra), Canoas campus, under the supervision of a qualified technician. The specimens were fixed in an artifact produced especially for the experiment (figure 9, page 38), in order to standardize their positioning and to allow the chisel of the testing machine to be directed exactly at the base of the brackets (figure 10, page 38).

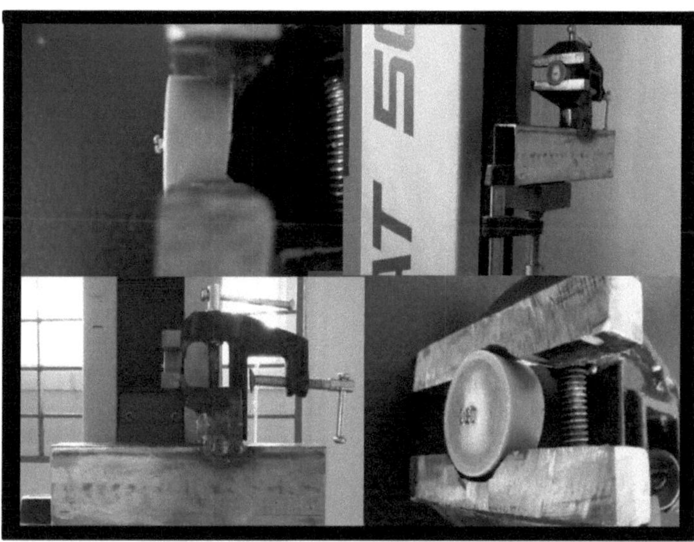

Figure 9 - Device built specifically for the experiment.

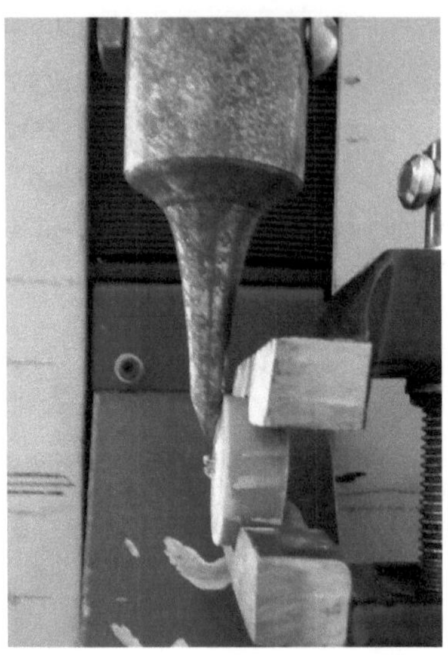

Figure 10 - Chisel aimed at the base of the briquette

The shear force was produced by a Versat Model 502M testing machine (Panambra Industrial e Tècnica S/A, Sâo Paulo, SP, Brazil) with a 500N (50 kgf) load cell (figure 11, page 39) and a speed of 0.5 mm/minute.

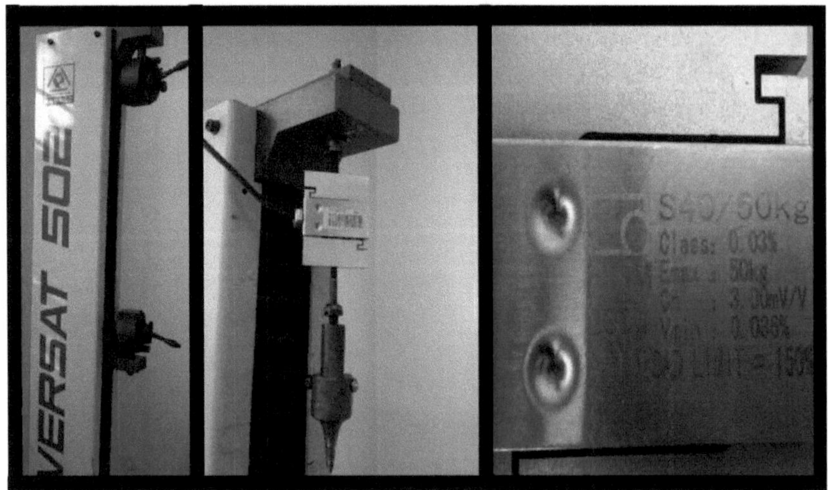

Figure 11 - Testing machine with load cell and chisel. On the right is a detail of the load cell.

When the bracket is detached from the tooth surface, the maximum shear force is entered in Newton (N) and automatically converted to shear stress in Megapascals (MPa) by dividing the load value (N) by the area of the bracket base (15.13 mm).^{2}

Tc = F/A, where:

Tc = shear stress (MPa); F = applied force (N); A = area of the flange (mm2).

The data in Megapascals (MPa) were tabulated for later statistical analysis.

4.6 - Adhesive Remnant Index (ARI) - in order to assess where the adhesion failure occurred, whether on the enamel surface, inherent to the resin itself or in the retentive area of the bracket, the Adhesive Remnant Index (ARI) recommended by Artun and Bergland in 1984 was used. The fracture areas were determined after the brackets were removed from the testing machine by a duly blinded and calibrated operator. The orthodontic brackets and teeth were observed using a 10X magnifying glass.

This index, shown in Table 7 below, establishes scores from 0 to 3 according to the amount of resin remaining on the enamel surface after the brackets have been removed.

Table 7 - Remaining adhesive index.

Index	Features
0	Absence of resin in the enamel
1	Less than 50% resin remaining on the tooth
2	More than 50% resin remaining on the tooth
3	Any remaining resin on the tooth

4.7 - Statistical treatment

Sample size calculation - assuming a statistical power of 80% (β=0.20) to detect a difference of one standard deviation between the means of at least two groups (E/S=1.0), it was estimated that 17 experimental units would be needed per group (total = 68 units) at a two-sided significance level of α/2=0.05. To compensate for any losses, 90 units were included in the study.

Statistical analysis - the quantitative shear force data was described by mean and standard deviation. The groups were compared using a one-way and two-way analysis of variance (ANOVA) model, with differences identified using the Student-Newman-Keuls (SNK) post-hoc test at a significance level (α=0.05). To compare ARI values, we used median and mean data and compared the groups using the Kruskal-Wallis test followed by Dunn's post-hoc procedure. To assess the correlation between shear forces and ARI, Spearman's correlation coefficient was calculated and its respective statistical significance by Student's t-test. The data was analyzed using SPSS version 22 and R version 3.3.0.

Calibration of the ARI operator - the ARI test was carried out by a blinded and properly calibrated operator. The operator's calibration was assessed using the Kappa coefficient, after three measurements of ten specimens with a one-day interval between each one. The Kappa values indicated high reproducibility of the evaluations, with 0.861 for the intervals from T1 to T2 and 1 for the intervals from T2 to T3.

5 - RESULTS

The mean, maximum, minimum, standard deviation and median values for the shear forces are shown in table 1 and graph 1 on page 44. The highest mean values were observed in the groups in which Optibond S (ethanol-based) adhesive was used, regardless of whether the teeth were bleached or not. The latter were higher than the former, 12.21 MPa ± 2.37 and 10.41 MPa ± 2.73, respectively. In the groups in which the adhesive chosen was Prime&Bond 2.1 (ketone-based), the average values were very similar in the bleached and unbleached groups, 8.89 MPa ± 2.16 and 8.48 MPa ± 1.53 respectively. The standard deviation observed is in the range of 20 to 50%, which is in line with the ISO/TS 11405:2015 standard for tests of adhesion to tooth structure.

Table 1 - Distribution of Shear Forces in MPa

Groups	N	Average	Deviation Standard	Median	Minimum	Maximum
1. Unbleached control and Prime& Bond 2.1	20	8,48 a	1,53	8,22	6,15	12,38
2. Unbleached control and Optibond S	21	12,21 b	2,37	12,36	7,40	16,95
3. Experimental bleached and Prime & Bond 2.1	20	8,89 a	2,16	8,62	5,17	15,49
4. Experimental bleached and Optibond S	21	10,41 c	2,73	10,83	4,98	14,95

p<0.001; non-coinciding index letters represent a statistically significant difference in the Student-Newman-Keuls SNK test (P<0.05)

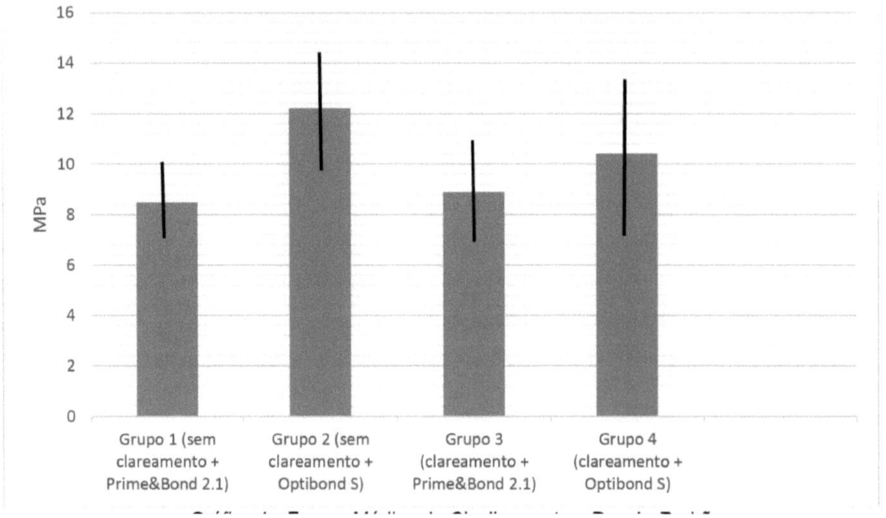

Graph 1 - Average Shear Forces and Standard Deviation

The groups were compared using one-way and two-way ANOVA analysis of variance to determine whether the differences were statistically significant. As shown in Table 2 below:

Table 2 - Analysis of Variance ANOVA

Variation source	Degrees of freedom	Sum of squares	Mean square	Test statistic f	Value -p
Groups	3	176,599	58,866	11,589	0,000
Error	78	396,194	5,079		
Total	81	572,794			

The ANOVA results indicate significant differences between the various groups (p 0.000).

The Student-Newman-Keuls post-hoc test was used to compare the groups, table 3 on page 45:

Table 3 - Student-Newman-Keuls test

Alpha = 0.05

Group	N	1	2	3

Student-Newman-Keuls	1a	20	8,4805		
	3a	20	8,8975		
	4b	21		10,4133	
	2c	21			12,2105
	Sig.		0,555	1,000	1,000

Unequal group sizes, used harmonic mean of sample size = 20.488 p<0.001; non-coinciding index letters represent statistically significant difference in SNK test (P<0.05)

G1 - Unbleached control group using Prime&Bond 2.1 adhesive

G2 - Unbleached control group using Optibond S adhesive

G3 - Bleached experimental group using Prime&Bond 2.1 adhesive G4 - Bleached experimental group using Optibond S adhesive

Statistically significant differences between the groups can be seen in table 4 on page 46. In the control groups, i.e. unbleached teeth, the shear forces for Optibond S adhesive were higher than those for Prime&Bond 2.1 (group 1 x 2). Shear forces on teeth that had been bleached using Optibond S adhesive were also higher than those for the unbleached group and Prime&Bond 2.1 adhesive (group 1 x 4). Again, the shear forces of Optibond S adhesive, now for unbleached teeth, were higher than the forces of bleached teeth using Prime&Bond 2.1 (group 2 x 3). The same can be said for the two groups that used Optibond S adhesive, regardless of bleaching or not (group 2 x 4). Finally, among the bleached groups, there was a significant difference between Optibond S and Prime&Bond 2.1 (group 3 x 4). No significant difference was found between the two groups that used Prime&Bond 2.1, whether the teeth were whitened or not (group 1 x 3).

Table 4 - Comparison between groups with Student-Newman-Keuls test

Comparisons	p-value
G1 X G2	<0,001
G1 X G3	0,56
G1 X G4	0,020
G2 X G3	<0,001
G2 X G4	0,013
G3 X G4	0,034

G1 - Unbleached control group using Prime&Bond 2.1 adhesive

G2 - Unbleached control group using Optibond S adhesive

The mean, maximum, minimum, standard deviation and median values for the Adhesive Remnant Index (ARI) are shown in Table 5. Median 2 was the same for all four groups. In the control groups without bleaching, regardless of the adhesive, the ARI ranged from 1 to 3. For the bleached experimental groups, if the adhesive used was Prime & Bond 2.1, the ARI ranged from 1 to 2 and if it was Optibond S, from 2 to 3.

Table 5 - Distribution of ARI Remaining Adhesive Index scores

Groups	N	Average	Deviation Standard	Median	Minimum	Maximo
Non-cleared control and Prime& Bond 2.1	20	1,85	0,59	2	1	3
Unbleached control and Optibond S	21	2,05	0,5	2	1	3
Experimental whitening and Prime & Bond 2.1	20	1,65	0,49	2	1	2
Experimental bleached and Optibond S	21	2,29	0,46	2	2	3

ARI scores

0 = no adhesive on the enamel

1= less than 50% adhesive on the enamel

2= more than 50% adhesive on the enamel

3= all the adhesive on the enamel

The groups were compared using the Kruskal-Wallis test. This indicated an overall p-value of 0.00195, table 6, indicating that there was at least one statistically significant difference between the groups.

Table 6 - Frequency of distribution of ARI scores (%)

Groups		ARI index				Total
		0	1	2	3	
1. Unbleached control and Prime& Bond 2.1	N	0	5	13	2	20

	%	0%	25%	65%	10%	100%
2. Unbleached control and Optibond S	N	0	2	16	3	21
	%	0%	9,5%	76,1%	14,2%	100%
3. Experimental bleached and Prime & Bond 2.1	N	0	7	13	0	20
	%	0%	35%	65%	0%	100%
4. Experimental bleached and Optibond S	N	0	0	15	6	21
	%	0%	0%	71,4%	28,7%	100%
Total	N	0	14	57	11	82

p = 0.00195 Kruskal-Wallis test

Dunn's test was then used to compare pairs of groups, table 7. This test reported a statistically significant difference in ARI between the Prime & Bond 2.1 and Optibond S groups in bleached teeth (groups 3 and 4), with a p-value of 0.0014. Thus, in the bleached groups, more resin remained on the enamel when Optibond S adhesive was used than when Prime & Bond 2.1 was used.

Table 7 - Dunn's test for comparing groups of ARI values

Group Comparison	p-values
unbleached Prime & Bond 2.1 X unbleached Optibond S (group 1 X group 2)	0,25
unbleached Prime & Bond 2.1 X bleached Prime & Bond 2.1 (group 1 X group 3)	0,25
unbleached Prime & Bond 2.1 X bleached Optibond S (group 1 X group 4)	0,053
unbleached Optibond S X bleached Prime & Bond 2.1 (group 2 X group 3)	0,085
unbleached Optibond S X bleached Optibond S (group 2 X group 4)	0,25
Prime & Bond 2.1 bleached X Optibond S bleached (group 3 X group 4)	0,0014*

* $p<0.05$ statistically significant

To assess the correlation between the variables shear strength and ARI, Spearman's correlation coefficient (r_s) was calculated and their respective statistical significance using Student's t-test. Scatter plots were also constructed for each group showing these two variables organized in relation to each other.

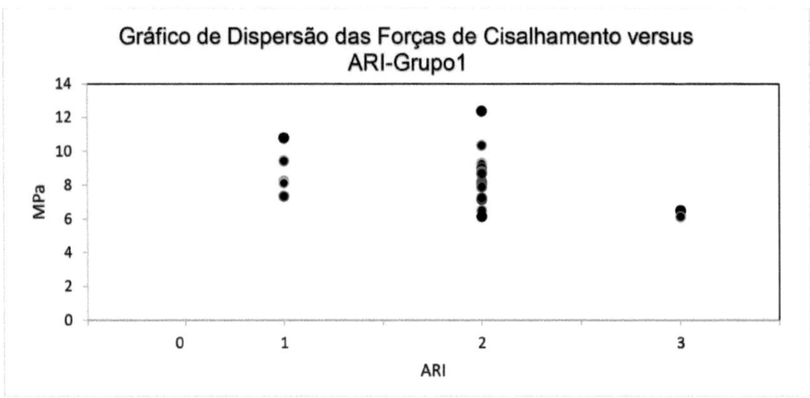

Graph 2 - Dispersion of Group 1

r_s = - 0,39p   = 0,086

Group 1 - unbleached control group using Prime&Bond 2.1 adhesive

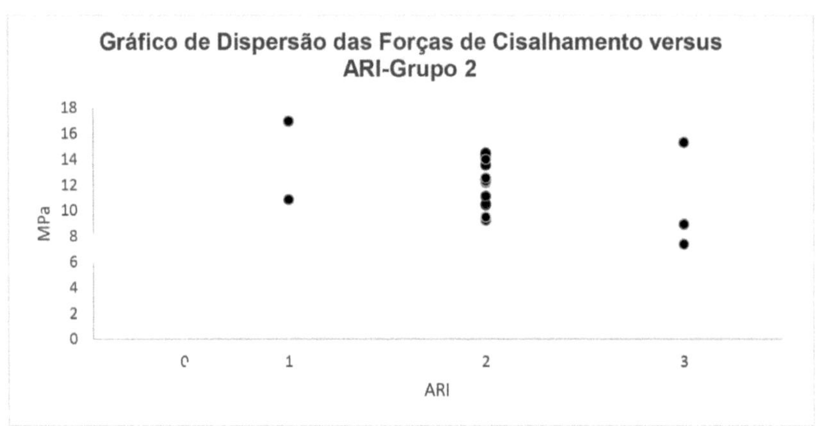

Graph 3 - Dispersion of Group 2

r_s = - 0,26p   = 0,26

Group 2 - unbleached control group using Optibond S adhesive

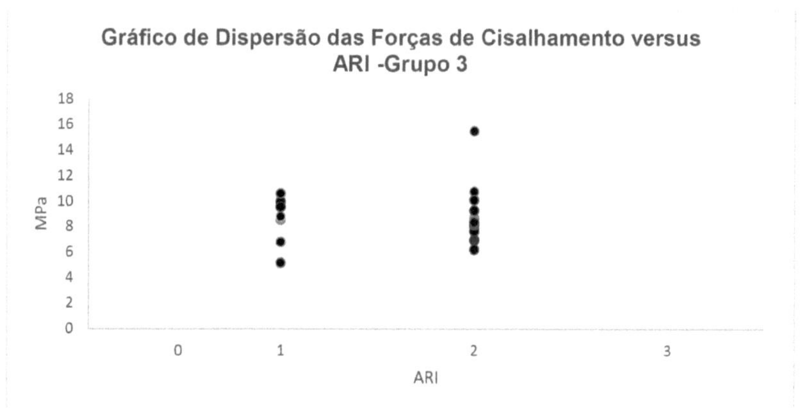

Graph 4 - Dispersion of Group 3

$r_s = 0.01$p $= 0.97$

Group 3 - experimental group bleached using Prime&Bond 2.1 adhesive

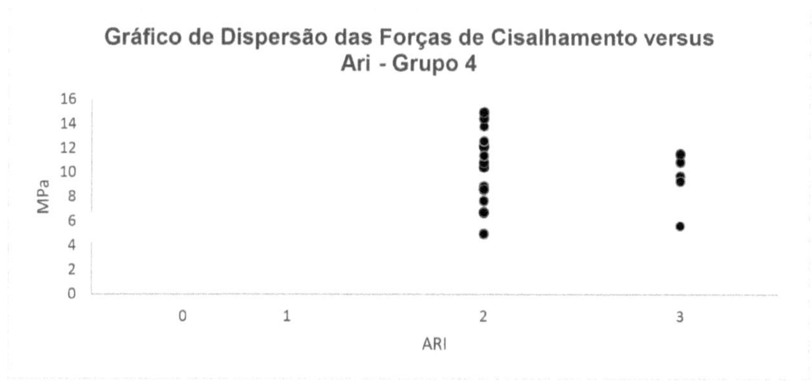

Graph 5 - Dispersion of Group 4

$r_s = - 0,24$p $= 0,29$

Group 4 - experimental group bleached using Optibond S adhesive

There was a weak correlation between shear force and ARI in groups 2, 3 and 4. Spearman's correlation coefficient (r_s) was between 0.1 and 0.3 for these three groups. In group 1, as ARI increased, shear force decreased moderately ($r_s = - 0.39$), a possible negative correlation.

6 - DISCUSSION

When we compared the mean shear force of the two bleached groups (groups 3 and 4) 9.67 MPa with the mean force of the two groups without bleaching (groups 1 and 2) 10.39 MPa, we obtained a non-significant difference (p=0.170). In agreement with the studies by Bishara et al. (2005) and Uysal et al. (2003). For them, bleaching does not affect the quality of adhesion.

When comparing the effect of the two adhesives on shear forces, we had different findings. The shear forces observed in the groups using Optibond (ethanol-based) were higher than those using Prime&Bond 2.1 (acetone-based). The average shear force for the two groups using Prime & Bond 2.1 adhesive (groups 1 and 3) was 8.69 MPa. For the two Optibond S adhesive groups (groups 2 and 4), it was 11.31 MPa. A highly significant difference (p<0.001). These findings are in line with those of Sung et al. (1999) and Shinohara et al. (2004). The first authors state that ethanol interacts with the residual oxygen in the whitening gel and minimizes the inhibitory effect of the whitening process on the formation of resin tags. Thus, the tags are better structured and longer, with greater adhesion to the tooth structure. They also state that ethanol-based adhesives can be used immediately after bleaching. Is it possible to say that Optibond S is superior to Prime & Bond 2.1? What is the clinical relevance of this finding? The lowest average shear forces in this study, observed in group 1, were still higher than the minimum values required for a bracket throughout orthodontic treatment according to the classic work by Reynolds (1975). On the other hand, the higher shear forces observed in the Optibond S groups could create a problem for the clinician when detaching the appliance once treatment is complete. The enamel could be damaged or fractured. Further scanning electron microscopy and surface roughness studies are needed to evaluate the enamel and compare the effects of the two adhesives.

For the Prime & Bond 2.1 groups (group 1 x group 3) there was no significant difference in shear strength. For the Optibond S adhesive groups (group 2 x group 4), there was a statistically significant difference between the bleached and unbleached groups. The difference was significant in the control groups (group 1 x group 2) and also in the bleached groups (group 3 x group 4). In the comparisons between the bleached group and Optibond S adhesive versus the unbleached group and Prime&Bond 2.1 adhesive (group 1 x group 4), there was a significant difference. There was also a significant difference between the unbleached group using Optibond S versus the bleached group using Prime&Bond 2.1 (group 2 x group 3).

The lowest average shear forces observed in this study were in group 1 (unbleached control using Prime&Bond 2.1 adhesive). They had a mean value of 8.22 MPa with a standard deviation of 1.53. These figures are even higher than the minimum values required for an orthodontic bracket to withstand chewing and orthodontic mechanics, according to studies by Reynolds (1975). For him, a bonding force of 6 to 8 MPa is the minimum required.

The changes in behavior in the presence of bleaching were more intense in the Optibond S groups than in the Prime&Bond 2.1 groups. The acetone-based adhesive was less affected by bleaching, as the shear strength showed no difference between bleached and unbleached teeth (groups 1 x 3). Some experiments report that acetone eliminates tooth surface moisture, the "water chaser" effect (BENNI, D. et al., 2014; NIAT, A. B. et al., 2012; NOUR EL-DIN et al., 2006; SWIFT, E. J. et al., 1999). However, although the ethanol-based adhesive suffered the greatest effect from bleaching, the lower shear bond strength among the groups using Optibond S (group 4) was still higher than the Prime&Bond 2.1 group with the highest bond strength (group 3).

Based on these findings, it is not possible to say that bleaching does not affect bonding forces. What can be said is that the 24-hour interval between the end of bleaching with 10% carbamide peroxide and the bonding of the orthodontic appliance is sufficient to safely assemble the appliance, regardless of whether the adhesive used is ethanol-based or acetone-based. This is in agreement with the studies by Martins (2008), Dishmann et al. (1994) and Titley et al. (1992).

The purpose of the Adhesive Remnant Index (ARI) is to inform where the adhesion failure occurred, whether in the enamel, inherent to the resin, or in the base of the bracket. Scores 1 and 2 clarify that the adhesion failures were inherent to the bonding resin, ruling out the poor quality of the retaining mesh of the bracket used, which would be informed by score 3. Finally, score 0 would indicate some problem in the enamel, such as a deleterious effect of bleaching. The mean scores for groups 1, 2, 3 and 4 were sequentially: 1.85 ± 0.59; 2.05 ± 0.5; 1.65 ± 0.49; 2.29 ± 0.46. These findings are in line with Heringer (2007). What is striking is that in none of the groups was a score of "0" found, which indicates that there was no resin remaining on the enamel after peeling. This score would be expected if acid etching failed or if bleaching had a detrimental effect on the adhesion quality of the brackets. The absence of a zero score, combined with the mean shear strength values obtained in the bleached groups, may suggest that the 24-hour interval between the end of bleaching with 10% carbamide peroxide in the home protocol and the bonding of the orthodontic appliance is sufficient. Of course, it cannot be ruled out that a longer time interval could provide even greater shear strength, but it is possible to infer that it is not necessary to wait two, three or four weeks as indicated by several authors (MULLINS, A. et al., 2009; GUNGOR, A.Y. et al., 2013; NASCIMENTO, G.C.R. et al., 2013). There was no significant difference in ARI between bleached and unbleached teeth. The same was observed by Cacciafesta et al. (2006) and Turkkahraman et al. (2007). Still in relation to ARI, the only statistically significant difference between the groups was for the two whitening groups. The score was higher for Optibond S compared to Prime&Bond 2.1 (group 3 vs. group 4). More resin was left on the enamel in the Optibond S group at the time of debonding. Once again the clinical question arises: is Optibond S superior to Prime&Bond 2.1 when bonding brackets 24 hours after bleaching? The fact that more adhesive has remained on the enamel may require more chair time to remove the remaining resin, which is obviously not an advantage.

The only correlation between shear strength and ARI was obtained in group 1, teeth that had not been bleached using Prime&Bond 2.1. Even so, it was a moderate correlation, according to Spearman's correlation coefficient. As the ARI increased, the shear force decreased. This is therefore a possible negative correlation: when an increase in one variable leads to a tendency for the other to decrease, but there may be other factors involved. For the other groups (2, 3 and 4) the correlation was small according to this coefficient. These findings are in line with the studies by Penido et al. (2008).

The different methodologies used in the studies described make it impossible to compare them. They differ in the type of tooth used, human vs. bovine, bleaching gel and its concentration, bleaching protocol, time between the end of bleaching and the bonding of the brackets, preparation of the specimens, means of storing them between bleaching sessions, inherent to the shear test itself (chisel activation speed, load cell used, specimen fixation device). When all the studies comply with the technical standards recommended for tests of adhesion to the tooth structure in ISO/TS 11405:2015, it will be possible to compare them.

Bovine incisors were used in this study. Bovine teeth have slightly lower adhesion forces, without statistical significance, than those observed in human teeth, provided that the principles of handling, storage and preparation are followed (NAKAMICHI, I. et al., 1983).

Carbamide peroxide at 10%, following the home protocol, is safer than the powerful hydrogen peroxide at 35% of the more traditional concentrations used in the office. Its effect is proven, perhaps slower, always respecting the particularities of each case, with less risk of gum irritation and hypersensitivity. For this reason, carbamide peroxide is the safest alternative and is recommended by the American Dental Association ADA (ALQAHTANI, M. Q., 2014; MARTINS, M. M., 2008; HERINGER, T. P., 2007).

This is an "in vitro" experimental study. Its findings and conclusions should therefore be viewed with caution. Clinical studies are essential to compare the effects of acetone- and ethanol-based adhesives on the bonding of orthodontic brackets on bleached or unbleached teeth.

7 - CONCLUSIONS

1)   There was no statistically significant difference in shear strength between control and bleached teeth in the 24-hour interval between the end of home bleaching with 10% carbamide peroxide and the bonding of the brackets;

2)   The time interval of 24 hours after home bleaching with 10% carbamide peroxide is sufficient for bonding orthodontic brackets;

3)   All the groups tested showed clinically acceptable bond strengths;

4)   The ethanol-based adhesive Optibond S had higher bond strengths than the acetone-based adhesive Prime&Bond 2.1 for both bleached and unbleached teeth;

5)   Optibond S adhesive had a higher ARI score than Prime&Bond 2.1 for bleached teeth, so more resin was left on the enamel at peeling when the ethanol-based adhesive was applied;

8 - BIBLIOGRAPHIC REFERENCES

ALQAHTANI, MQ. Tooth-bleaching procedures and their controversial effects: A literature review. Saudi dent. j. 2014;26(2): 33-46.

ARTUN, J, BERGLAND, S. Clinical trials with crystal growth conditioning as an alternative to acid-etch enamel pretreatment. Am. j. orthod. 1984;85(4):333-40.

BELO, DRM, SOUZA, MAL. The influence of tooth whitening, *in vitro,* on the bonding of *brackets* with resin-modified glass ionomer cement. Ortodon. gaùch. 2000;4(2): 87-100.

BENNI, D et al. An in vitro study to evaluate the effect of two ethanol-based and two acetone-based dental bonding agents on the bond strength of composite to enamel treated with 10% carbamide peroxide. J. Indian Soc. Pedod. Prev. Dent. 2014;32(3): 207-11.

BISHARA, SE et al. The effect of tooth bleaching on the shear bond strength of orthodontic brackets. Am. j. orthod. dentofacial orthop. 2005;128(6): 755-60.

BULUT, H et al. Effect of an antioxidying agent on the shear bond strength of brackets bonded to bleached human enamel. Am. j. orthod. dentofacial orthop. 2006;129(2): 266-72.

CACCIAFESTA, V et al. The effect of bleaching on the shear bond strength of brackets bonded with a resin-modified glass ionomer. Am. j. orthod. dentofacial orthop. 2006;130(1):83-7.

DELLA BONA, A; GUIDA, LA. Scientific evidence for the adhesion of ceramic brackets to different dental substrates. Salusvita 2014; 33(3): 365-87.

FARRET, MM et al. Influence of methodological variables on shear bond strength. Rev. dent. press ortodon. ortop. facial. 2010; 15(1): 80-8.

FINNEMA, KJ et al. In-vitro orthodontic bond strength testing: A systematic review and meta-analysis. Am. j. orthod. dentofacial orthop. 2010; 137(5):615- 22.

GUNGOR, AY et al. Effects of different bleaching methods on shear strengths of orthodontic brackets. Angle orthod. 2013;83(4): 686-90.

HERINGER, TP. Influence of the use of teeth whitening agents on the adhesion of orthodontic brackets. [Dissertation] Belo Horizonte (MG): Pontificia Universidade Católica de Minas Gerais; 2007.

ISO/TS 11405:2015. Dentistry -Testing of adhesion to tooth structure. p 12. Gen- ebra, Switzerland.

JOINER, A. The bleaching of the teeth: a review of the literature. J. dent. 2006;34,(7): 412-9.

KNOSEL, M et al. External bleaching effect on the color and luminosity of inactive white-spot lesions after fixed orthodontic appliances. Angle orthod. 2007;77(4): 646-52.

KRAETHER, J, SOUZA, MAL. The influence of in vitro tooth whitening on bracket bonding. Ortodon. gaùch. 2002;6(1): 6-16.

MARTINS, MM. Influência dos procedimentos de clareamento dental na adesâo de acessórios ortodonticos.[Dissertaçâo] Rio de Janeiro (RJ): Universidade do Estado do Rio de Janeiro; 2008.

MONTALVAN, E et al. The shear bond strength of acetone and ethanol-based bonding agents to bleached teeth. Pediatr. dent. 2006;28(6): 531-6.

MULLINS, A et al. Tooth whitening effects on bracket bond strength in vivo. Angle orthod. 2009;79(4): 777-83.

NAKAMICHI, I et al. Bovine teeth as possible substitutes in the adhesion test. J. dent. res. 1983;62(10): 1076-81.

NASCIMENTO, GCR. et al. Does the time interval after bleaching influence the adhesion of orthodontic brackets? Korean. j. orthod. 2013;43(5): 242-7.

NIAT, AB et al. Effects of Drying Agents on Bond Strength of Etch-and-Rinse Adhesive

Systems to Enamel Immediately after Bleaching. J. adhes. dent. 2012;14(6): 511-6.

NOUR EL-DIN, et al. Immediated Bonding to Bleached Enamel. Oper. dent. 2006;31(1): 106-14.

PATUSCO, VC et al. Bond strength of metallic brackets after dental bleaching. Angle orthod. 2009;79(1): 122-6.

PENIDO, SMMO et al. In vivo and in vitro study, with and without thermocycling, of the shear bond strength of brackets bonded with a halogen light source. Rev. dent. press ortodon. ortop. facial. 2008;13(3): 66-76.

PHAN, X et al. Effect of tooth bleaching on shear strength of a fluoride releasing sealant. Angle orthod. 2012;82(3): 546-51.

PRIETSCH, JR et al. Influence of tooth whitening with hydrogen peroxide on orthodontic bracket bonding: an in vitro study. Ortodon. gaùch. 2003;7(2): 136-44.

REYNOLDS, IR. A review of direct orthodontic bonding. Br. j. orthod. 1975;138(2): 171-8.

SCOUGALL-VILCHIS, RJ et al. Influence of four systems for dental bleaching on the bond strength of orthodontic brackets. Angle orthod. 2011;81(4): 700-6.

SHINOHARA, MS et al. The effect of non-vital bleaching on the shear bond strength of composite resin using three adhesive systems. J. adhes. dent. 2004;6(3):205-9.

SUNG, EC et al. Effect of carbamide peroxide bleaching on the shear bond strength of composite dental bonding agent enhanced enamel. J. prosthet. dent. 1999;82(1): 595-9.

SWIFT, EJ et al. Shear Bond Strengths of One-Bottle Adhesives to Moist Enamel. J. esthet. restor. dent. 1999;11(2): 103-107.

TUKKAHRAMAN, H et al. Bleaching and Desensitizer application effects on shear bond strengths of orthodontic brackets. Angle orthod. 2007;77(3): 489-93.

UYSAL, T et al. Can previously bleached teeth be bonded safely? Am. j. orthod. dentofacial orthop. 2003;123(6): 628-32.

UYSAL, T, SISMAN, A. Can previously bleached teeth be bonded safely using self-etching primer systems? Angle orthod. 2008;78(4): 711-5.

YADALA, C et al. Comparison of Shear Bond Strength of Three Self-etching Adhesives: an In-vitro Study. J. int. oral health. 2015;7(7): 53-7.

YADAV, D et al. Effect of tooth bleaching on orthodontic stainless steel bracket bond strength. J. orthod. science. 2015;4(3): 72-6.

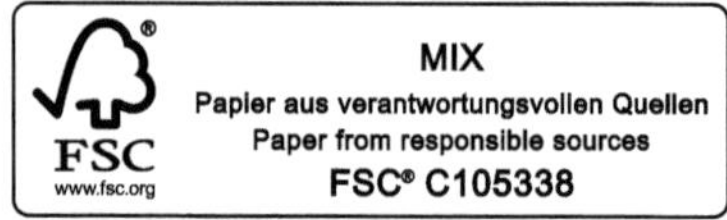

Printed by Books on Demand GmbH, Norderstedt / Germany